100 Arthritis Meal and Juice Recipes:

Naturally Reduce Pain and Discomfort

By

Joe Correa CSN

COPYRIGHT

This publication is designed to provide accurate and authoritative information in regard to the subject matter covered. It is sold with the understanding that neither the author nor the publisher is engaged in rendering medical advice. If medical advice or assistance is needed, consult with a doctor. This book is considered a guide and should not be used in any way detrimental to your health. Consult with a physician before starting this nutritional plan to make sure it's right for you.

ACKNOWLEDGEMENTS

This book is dedicated to my friends and family that have had mild or serious illnesses so that you may find a solution and make the necessary changes in your life.

100 Arthritis Meal and Juice Recipes:

Naturally Reduce Pain and Discomfort

By

Joe Correa CSN

CONTENTS

Copyright

Acknowledgements

About The Author

Introduction

100 Arthritis Meal and Juice Recipes: Naturally Reduce Pain and Discomfort

Additional Titles from This Author

ABOUT THE AUTHOR

After years of Research, I honestly believe in the positive effects that proper nutrition can have over the body and mind. My knowledge and experience has helped me live healthier throughout the years and which I have shared with family and friends. The more you know about eating and drinking healthier, the sooner you will want to change your life and eating habits.

Nutrition is a key part in the process of being healthy and living longer so get started today. The first step is the most important and the most significant.

INTRODUCTION

100 Arthritis Meal and Juice Recipes: Naturally Reduce Pain and Discomfort

By Joe Correa CSN

There are about 100 different types of arthritis, but the most common ones are rheumatoid arthritis and osteoarthritis. Unlike rheumatoid arthritis which is an autoimmune disorder, osteoarthritis is described as a degenerative joint disease. The exact cause of arthritis is unknown, but there are many different factors that may affect the autoimmune response, including genetic susceptibility. Early symptoms for both types include painful swelling of joints, morning stiffness, and inflammation.

With a good nutrition, consistency, and good lifestyle choices, your health will improve significantly and your body will get a chance to resist the inflammation you feel when you have arthritis. Furthermore, healthy, fresh, and unprocessed foods will reduce the risk of obesity which not only contributes to the onset and progress of arthritis but also makes your joints carry more weight. Excess weight directly damages your joints and contributes to both - development and progress of this disease.

Juicing is one of the best ways to nourish your body with amazingly valuable antioxidants and other important substances in just a few minutes. This collection of juice and meal recipes is especially practical for people with busy schedules who have very little to prepare everything.

These recipes will make your digestion easier and will help eliminate dangerous toxins that lead to inflammation and arthritis. This book is a more convenient way to preventing arthritis once and for all no matter what your current situation is.

100 ARTHRITIS MEAL AND JUICE RECIPES: NATURALLY REDUCE PAIN AND DISCOMFORT

JUICE RECIPES

1.   Blueberry celery Juice

Ingredients:

2 cups of fresh blueberries

3 large stalks of celery, sliced

1 large lemon, peeled

1 medium-sized Granny smith apple, cored

2 oz of water

Preparation:

Using a colander, wash the blueberries under cold running water. Cut in half and remove the leaves. Set aside.

Wash the celery and cut into thick slices. Set aside.

Peel the lemon and cut lengthwise in half. Set aside.

Wash the apple and remove the core. Cut into bite-sized pieces and set aside.

Now, combine blueberries, celery, lemon, and apple in a juicer and process until juiced. Transfer to serving glasses and stir in the water. Add few ice cubes before serving.

Enjoy!

Nutritional information per serving: Kcal: 296, Protein: 6.6g, Carbs: 88.4g, Fats: 1.4g

2.   Orange Apricot Juice

Ingredients:

2 large oranges, peeled

2 large apricots, pitted

1 cup of pomegranate seeds

1 cup of green grapes

1 large lemon, peeled

1 small ginger slice, peeled

Preparation:

Peel the oranges and divide into wedges. Set aside.

Wash the apricots and cut in half. Remove the pits and cut into small pieces. Set aside.

Cut the top of the pomegranate fruit using a sharp knife. Slice down to each of the white membranes inside of the fruit. Pop the seeds into a measuring cup and set aside.

Peel the lemon and cut lengthwise in half. Set aside.

Peel the ginger slice and set aside.

Now, combine oranges, apricots, pomegranate, lemon, and ginger in a juicer. Process until well juiced and transfer to serving glasses. Refrigerate for 20 minutes before serving.

Nutritional information per serving: Kcal: 294, Protein: 7.2g, Carbs: 88.9g, Fats: 2.3g

3.   Blueberry Mint Juice

Ingredients:

1 cup of blueberries

1 cup of fresh mint, torn

1 large red apple, cored

1 large cucumber, sliced

2 oz of coconut water

Preparation:

Place the blueberries in a colander and wash under cold running water. Drain and set aside.

Wash the mint thoroughly and torn with hands. Set aside.

Wash the apple and cut in half. Remove the core and cut into bite-sized pieces. Set aside.

Wash the cucumber and gently peel it. Cut into thin slices and set aside.

Now, combine blueberries, mint, apple, and cucumber in a juicer. Process until juiced and transfer to serving glasses. Stir in the coconut water and refrigerate for 15 minutes, or add some ice before serving.

Enjoy!

Nutritional information per serving: Kcal: 258, Protein: 4.7g, Carbs: 74.6g, Fats: 1.6g

4.   Strawberry Mango Juice

Ingredients:

6 large strawberries, chopped

1 cup of mango, peeled and chopped

1 cup of cantaloupe, chopped

1 large cucumber, sliced

2 oz of coconut water

Preparation:

Wash the strawberries and cut into bite-sized pieces. Set aside.

Peel the mango and cut into small chunks. Fill the measuring cup and reserve the rest for later.

Cut the cantaloupe in half and scoop out the seeds. Cut two wedges and peel them. Chop into chunks and fill the measuring cup. Reserve the rest of the cantaloupe in a refrigerator.

Wash the cucumber and cut into thick slices. Set aside.

Now, combine strawberries, mango, cantaloupe, and cucumber in a juicer and process until juiced. Transfer to serving glasses and stir in the coconut water. refrigerate for 30 minutes before serving.

Enjoy!

Nutritional information per serving: Kcal: 209, Protein: 5.3g, Carbs: 56.6g, Fats: 1.5g

5.   Avocado Citrus Juice

Ingredients:

1 cup of avocado, pitted and chopped

1 large cucumber, sliced

1 large lemon, peeled

1 cup of fresh spinach, torn

1 large lime, peeled

1 small ginger knob, peeled

3 oz of water

Preparation:

Peel the avocado and cut in half. Remove the pit and chop into chunks. Set aside.

Wash the cucumber and cut into thick slices. Set aside.

Peel the lemon and lime. Cut lengthwise in half and set aside.

Wash the spinach thoroughly and torn with hands. Set aside.

Peel the ginger knob and set aside.

Now, combine avocado, cucumber, lemon, lime, spinach, and ginger in a juicer. Process until juiced and transfer to serving glasses. Stir in the water and refrigerate for 20 minutes before serving.

Enjoy!

Nutritional information per serving: Kcal: 269, Protein: 6.7g, Carbs: 35g, Fats: 22.6g

6. Artichoke Turmeric Juice

Ingredients:

1 large artichoke, peeled and chopped

1 cup of Brussels sprouts, trimmed

1 large carrot, sliced

1 cup of fresh celery, chopped

1 cup of turnip greens, chopped

1 large green apple, cored

½ tsp of turmeric, ground

2 oz of water

Preparation:

Using a sharp knife, trim off the outer leaves of the artichoke. Cut into small pieces and set aside.

Trim off the outer leaves of the Brussels sprouts and wash them thoroughly. Cut in half and set aside.

Wash the carrot and cut into thin slices. Set aside.

Wash the celery and chop it into bite-sized pieces. Set aside.

Wash the apple and cut in half. Remove the core and cut into bite-sized pieces. Set aside.

Wash the turnip greens thoroughly and torn with hands. Set aside.

Now, combine artichoke, Brussels sprouts, carrot, celery, turnip greens, and apple in a juicer. Process until well juiced and transfer to serving glasses. Stir in the turmeric and water. Add some ice before serving.

Nutritional information per serving: Kcal: 205, Protein: 11.3g, Carbs: 66.7g, Fats: 1.4g

7.   Watermelon Orange Juice

Ingredients:

2 cups of watermelon, chopped

1 large orange, peeled

1 cup of raspberries

1 large kiwi, peeled

2 oz coconut water

Preparation:

Cut the watermelon lengthwise. For 2 cups, you will need about 2 large wedges. Peel and cut into chunks. Remove the seeds and set aside. Reserve the rest of the melon for some other juices. Set aside.

Peel the orange and divide into wedges. Set aside.

Wash the raspberries thoroughly under cold running water. Drain and set aside.

Peel the kiwi and cut lengthwise in half. Set aside.

Now, combine watermelon, orange, raspberries, and kiwi in a juicer. Process until juiced and transfer to serving glasses. Stir in the coconut water and refrigerate for 15 minutes before serving.

Nutritional information per serving: Kcal: 232, Protein: 5.8g, Carbs: 71.4g, Fats: 1.8g

8.   Salted Beet Tomato Juice

Ingredients:

2 cups of beets, trimmed

1 large Roma tomato, chopped

1 large cucumber, sliced

3 large radishes, trimmed

½ tsp of fresh rosemary, chopped

¼ tsp of sea salt

1 oz of water

Preparation:

Wash the beets and trim off the green parts. Cut into small pieces and set aside.

Wash the tomato and place it in a bowl. Cut into bite-sized pieces and reserve the tomato juice while cutting. Set aside.

Wash the cucumber and cut into thin slices. Set aside.

Wash the radishes and trim off the green ends. Cut in half and set aside.

Now, combine beets, tomato, cucumber, radishes, and rosemary in a juicer. Process until well juiced and transfer to serving glasses. Stir in the salt and water. refrigerate for 10 minutes before serving.

Enjoy!

Nutritional information per serving: Kcal: 152, Protein: 8.2g, Carbs: 44.9g, Fats: 1.2g

9.   Pepper Squash Juice

Ingredients:

3 large red bell peppers, chopped

1 cup of butternut squash, cubed

1 cup of parsnip, sliced

1 tbsp of fresh parsley, chopped

2 oz of water

Preparation:

Wash the red bell peppers and cut lengthwise in half. Remove the seeds and chop into small pieces.

Peel the butternut squash and remove the seeds using a spoon. Cut into small cubes and fill the measuring cup. Reserve the rest of the squash for some other recipe. Wrap in a plastic foil and refrigerate.

Wash the parsnip and peel it. Cut into thin slices and set aside.

Now, combine bell peppers, butternut squash, parsnip, and parsley in a juicer. Process until well juiced and transfer to serving glasses. Stir in the water and add some ice.

Serve immediately.

Nutritional information per serving: Kcal: 238, Protein: 7.9g, Carbs: 70.2g, Fats: 2.1g

10.   Papaya Pomegranate Juice

Ingredients:

1 large papaya, peeled and chopped

1 cup of pomegranate seeds

1 large green apple, cored

1 tbsp of fresh mint, chopped

2 oz of water

Preparation:

Peel the papaya and cut lengthwise in half. Scoop out the black seeds and flesh using a spoon. Cut into small chunks and set aside.

Cut the top of the pomegranate fruit using a sharp knife. Slice down to each of the white membranes inside of the fruit. Pop the seeds into a measuring cup and set aside.

Wash the apple and cut in half. Using a sharp knife, remove the core and cut into bite-sized pieces. Set aside.

Now, combine papaya, pomegranate, apple, and mint in a juicer. Process until well juiced and transfer to serving glasses. Stir in the water and refrigerate for 15 minutes before serving.

Nutritional information per serving: Kcal: 438, Protein: 6.1g, Carbs: 129g, Fats: 3.4g

11.   Plum Blackberry Juice

Ingredients:

5 large plums, pitted

2 cups of blackberries

1 large lemon, peeled

1 cup of black grapes

1 medium-sized Golden delicious apple, cored

2 oz of water

1 tsp of liquid honey

Preparation:

Wash the plums and cut in half. Remove the pits and cut in small pieces. Set aside.

Wash the blackberries thoroughly under cold running water. Drain and set aside.

Peel the lemon and cut lengthwise in half. Set aside.

Wash the black grapes and set aside.

Wash the apple and cut in half. Remove the core and cut into bite-sized pieces. Set aside.

Now, combine plums, blackberries, lemon, black grapes, and apple in a juicer. Process until well juiced and transfer to serving glasses. Stir in the honey and water. Add some ice and serve immediately.

Enjoy!

Nutritional information per serving: Kcal: 344, Protein: 8g, Carbs: 110g, Fats: 3.1g

12.   Pineapple Lime Juice

Ingredients:

1 cup of pineapple chunks

2 large limes, peeled

1 cup of guava, chopped

1 large cucumber, sliced

1 tbsp of fresh basil, chopped

2 oz of water

Preparation:

Cut the top of a pineapple and peel it using a sharp knife. Cut into small chunks and fill the measuring cup. Reserve the rest of the pineapple in a refrigerator.

Peel the limes and cut lengthwise in half. Set aside.

Wash the guava and cut into chunks. Fill the measuring cup and reserve the rest for some other recipe in a refrigerator.

Wash the cucumber and cut into thin slices. Set aside.

Now, combine pineapple, limes, guava, cucumber, and basil in a juicer. Process until well juiced and transfer to serving glasses. Stir in the water and refrigerate for 15 minutes before serving.

Nutritional information per serving: Kcal: 158, Protein: 4.7g, Carbs: 47.9g, Fats: 1.1g

13.   Cranberry Pear Juice

Ingredients:

1 cup of cranberries

1 large pear, cored

1 large green apple, cored

3 large strawberries, chopped

1 large orange, peeled

¼ tsp of nutmeg, ground

2 oz of coconut water

Preparation:

Wash the cranberries thoroughly under cold running water. Drain and set aside.

Wash the pear and cut lengthwise in half. Remove the core and cut into bite-sized pieces. Set aside.

Wash the apple and cut in half. Remove the core and cut into bite-sized pieces. Set aside.

Wash the strawberries thoroughly and chop into small pieces. Set aside.

Peel the orange and divide into wedges. Set aside.

Now, combine pear, apple, strawberries, orange, and nutmeg in a juicer. Process until well juiced and transfer to serving glasses. Stir in the water and refrigerate or add some ice before serving.

Nutritional information per serving: Kcal: 158, Protein: 4.7g, Carbs: 47.9g, Fats: 1.1g

14.　Carrot Orange Juice

Ingredients:

5 large carrots, peeled

1 large orange, peeled and wedged

1 large lemon, peeled

1 cup of Romaine lettuce, torn

1 large cucumber, sliced

¼ tsp of turmeric, ground

Preparation:

Peel and wash the carrots. Cut into thin slices and set aside.

Peel the orange and divide into wedges. Set aside.

Peel the lemon and cut lengthwise in half. Set aside.

Wash the lettuce thoroughly and torn with hands. Set aside.

Wash the cucumber and cut into thin slices. Set aside.

Now, combine carrots, orange, lemon, lettuce, and cucumber in a juicer. Process until well juiced and transfer to serving glasses. stir in the turmeric and add some ice before serving. Enjoy!

Nutritional information per serving: Kcal: 232, Protein: 8.2g, Carbs: 74g, Fats: 1.7g

15.   Asparagus Collard Greens Juice

Ingredients:

1 cup of asparagus, trimmed

1 cup of collard greens, torn

1 cup of watercress, torn

1 green bell pepper, chopped

1 large cucumber, sliced

2 oz of water

¼ tsp of salt

Preparation:

Wash the asparagus and trim off the woody ends. Cut into bite-sized pieces and fill the measuring cup. Reserve the rest for some other juice.

Combine collard greens and watercress in a colander. Wash thoroughly under cold running water and torn with hands. Set aside.

Wash the bell pepper and lengthwise in half. Remove the seeds and chop into small pieces. Set aside.

Wash the cucumber and cut into thin slices. Set aside.

Now, combine asparagus, collard greens, bell pepper, and cucumber in a juicer and process until well juiced. Transfer to serving glasses and stir in the salt and water. refrigerate for 15 minutes before serving.

Nutritional information per serving: Kcal: 86, Protein: 8.2g, Carbs: 26.1g, Fats: 1g

16. Sweet Potato Green Smoothie

Ingredients:

1 cup of sweet potatoes, peeled

1 large fennel, chopped

1 cup of Swiss chard, torn

1 cup of red leaf lettuce, torn

1 cup of fresh spinach, torn

1 small cauliflower head, chopped

1 large lemon, peeled

Preparation:

Peel the sweet potato and cut into small chunks. Fill the measuring cup and reserve the rest for some other juice.

Wash the fennel bulb and trim off the wilted outer layers. Cut into small chunks and set aside.

Combine Swiss chard, red leaf lettuce, and spinach in a colander. Wash under cold running water and drain. Torn with hands and set aside.

Trim off the outer leaves of cauliflower. Wash it and cut into small pieces. Set aside.

Peel the lemon and cut lengthwise in half. Set aside.

Now, combine potato, fennel, Swiss chard, cauliflower, and lemon in a juicer and process until well juiced. Transfer to serving glasses and add some ice before serving.

Nutritional information per serving: Kcal: 218, Protein: 14.3g, Carbs: 67.7g, Fats: 1.9g

17.   Fennel Brussels Sprouts Juice

Ingredients:

1 medium-sized fennel bulb, chopped

1 cup of Brussels sprouts, halved

1 large yellow bell pepper, chopped

1 large cucumber, sliced

¼ tsp of salt

2 oz of water

Preparation:

Trimm off the fennel stalks and wilted outer layers. Cut into bite-sized pieces and set aside.

Trim off the outer leaves and wash the Brussels sprouts. Cut in half and set aside.

Wash the bell pepper and cut lengthwise in half. Remove the seeds and chop into small pieces. Set aside.

Wash the cucumber and cut into thin slices. Set aside.

Now, combine fennel, Brussels sprouts, bell peppers, and cucumber in a juicer. Process until well juiced and stir in the salt and water. Refrigerate for 10 minutes before serving.

Nutritional information per serving: Kcal: 151, Protein: 9.7g, Carbs: 47.6g, Fats: 1.4g

18.   Watermelon Peach Juice

Ingredients:

1 cup of watermelon, cubed

2 large peaches, pitted

1 large green apple, cored

5 fresh cherries, pitted

3 oz of coconut water

Preparation:

Cut the watermelon lengthwise. For one cup, you will need about one large wedge. Peel and cut into chunks. Remove the seeds and set aside. Reserve the rest of the melon for some other juices.

Wash the peaches and cut in half. Remove the pits and cut into bite-sized pieces. Set aside.

Wash the apple and cut in half. Remove the core and cut into bite-sized pieces. Set aside.

Wash the cherries and cut in half. Remove the pits and set aside.

Now, process watermelon, peaches, apple, and cherries in a juicer. Transfer to serving glasses and stir in the coconut water. Add some ice and serve immediately.

Nutritional information per serving: Kcal: 276, Protein: 5.4g, Carbs: 47.6g, Fats: 1.6g

19.   Spinach Apple Juice

Ingredients:

1 cup of fresh spinach, torn

1 large red apple, cored

1 cup of wild asparagus, trimmed

1 cup of collard greens, torn

1 cup of mustard greens, torn

2 oz of water

Preparation:

Combine spinach, collard greens, and mustard greens in a large colander. Wash under cold running water and drain. Torn with hands and set aside.

Wash the apple and cut in half. Remove the core and cut into bite-sized pieces. Set aside.

Now, combine spinach, collard greens, mustard greens, and apple in a juicer and process until well juiced. Transfer to serving glasses and stir in the water. refrigerate for 15 minutes before serving.

Nutritional information per serving: Kcal: 207, Protein: 16.1g, Carbs: 58.6g, Fats: 2.5g

20.   Plum Cabbage Juice

Ingredients:

5 large plums, pitted

1 cup of purple cabbage, chopped

1 cup of blackberries

1 large cucumber, sliced

2 oz of water

Preparation:

Wash the plums and cut in half. Remove the pits and cut into quarters. Set aside.

Wash the cabbage thoroughly under cold running water. Drain and roughly chop it. Set aside.

Wash the blackberries under cold running water using a colander. Slightly drain and set aside.

Wash the cucumber and cut into thin slices. Set aside.

Now, combine plums, cabbage, blackberries, and cucumber in a juicer and process until juice. Transfer to serving glasses and stir in the water. refrigerate for 15 minutes before serving.

Nutritional information per serving: Kcal: 221, Protein: 7.5g, Carbs: 69.1g, Fats: 2.1g

21.   Crookneck Squash Tomato Juice

Ingredients:

1 cup of crookneck squash, chopped

1 large tomato, chopped

1 large lemon, peeled

1 large orange, peeled

1 large pear, cored and chopped

2 oz of water

1 tsp of liquid honey

Preparation:

Wash the crookneck squash and cut in half. Scoop out the seeds using a spoon. Cut into small chunks and fill the measuring cup. Reserve the rest for another juice.

Wash the tomato and place it in a bowl. Cut into bite-sized pieces and reserve the juice while cutting. Set aside.

Peel the lemon and cut lengthwise in half. Set aside.

Peel the orange and divide into wedges. Set aside.

Wash the pear and cut lengthwise in half. Remove the core and cut into bite-sized pieces. Set aside.

Now, combine crookneck squash, tomato, lemon, orange, and pear in a juicer. Process until well juiced and transfer to serving glasses. Stir in the water and honey. Add some ice and serve immediately.

Nutritional information per serving: Kcal: 201, Protein: 5.9g, Carbs: 66.1g, Fats: 1.3g

22. Cauliflower Leek Juice

Ingredients:

1 small cauliflower head, chopped

3 large leeks, chopped

1 large lime, peeled

1 large zucchini, chopped

2 oz of water

Preparation:

Trim off the outer leaves of cauliflower. Wash it and cut into small pieces. Set aside.

Wash the leeks and cut into small pieces. Set aside.

Peel the lime and cut lengthwise in half. Set aside.

Peel the zucchini and cut in half. Scrape out the seeds and cut into small chunks. Set aside.

Now, combine cauliflower, leeks, lime, and zucchini in a juicer. Process until well juiced and stir in the water. Refrigerate for 10 minutes before serving.

Nutritional information per serving: Kcal: 241, Protein: 13.2g, Carbs: 64.7g, Fats: 2.6g

23.   Raspberry Beet Juice

Ingredients:

2 cups of raspberries

1 large green apple, cored

1 cup of beets, chopped

1 cup of fresh basil, torn

1 large lemon, peeled

3 oz of water

Preparation:

Wash the raspberries under cold running water using a colander. Drain and set aside.

Wash the apple and cut in half. Remove the core and cut into bite-sized pieces. Set aside.

Wash the beets and trim off the green ends. Cut into small pieces and fill the measuring cup. Reserve the greens for some other juice.

Wash the basil thoroughly under cold running water and torn with hands. Set aside.

Peel the lemon and cut lengthwise in half. Set aside.

Now, combine raspberries, apple, beets, basil, and lemon in a juicer. Process until well juiced. Stir in the water and refrigerate for 10 minutes before serving.

Enjoy!

Nutritional information per serving: Kcal: 218, Protein: 7.5g, Carbs: 76.4g, Fats: 2.5g

24.   Apricot Pomegranate Juice

Ingredients:

1 large apricot, pitted

1 cup of pomegranate seeds

1 large lemon, peeled

1 large orange, wedged

1 large carrot, peeled

2 oz of coconut water

Preparation:

Wash the apricot and cut in half. Remove the pit and cut into small pieces. Set aside.

Cut the top of the pomegranate fruit using a sharp knife. Slice down to each of the white membranes inside of the fruit. Pop the seeds into measuring cup and set aside.

Peel the lemon and cut lengthwise in half. Set aside.

Peel the orange and divide into wedges. Set aside.

Peel and wash the carrot. Cut into thin slices and set aside.

Now, combine apricot, pomegranate seeds, lemon, orange, and carrot in a juicer. Process until well juiced and transfer to serving glasses. Stir in the coconut water and add few ice cubes before serving.

Nutritional information per serving: Kcal: 241, Protein: 7.3g, Carbs: 73.9g, Fats: 2.3g

25. Broccoli Kale Juice

Ingredients:

2 cups of broccoli, trimmed

1 cup of fresh kale, torn

1 cup of fresh parsley, torn

1 large green apple, chopped

1 cup of fresh spinach, torn

2 oz of water

Preparation:

Wash the broccoli under cold running water and cut into small pieces. Set aside.

Combine parsley, kale, and spinach in a colander and wash under cold running water. Drain and torn with hands. Set aside.

Wash the apple and cut in half. Remove the core and cut into bite-sized pieces. Set aside.

Now, combine broccoli, kale, parsley, apple, and spinach in a juicer. Process until well juiced and stir in the water.

Refrigerate for 20 minutes before serving.

Nutritional information per serving: Kcal: 223, Protein: 20.4g, Carbs: 62.1g, Fats: 3.5g

26.   Mango Cherry Juice

Ingredients:

1 cup of mango, chopped

1 cup of fresh cherries, pitted

2 cup of green grapes

1 large lemon, peeled

2 oz of water

Preparation:

Wash the mango and cut into chunks. Fill the measuring cup and reserve the rest for some other juice. Set aside.

Wash the cherries and cut in half. Remove the pits and set aside.

Wash the grapes and fill the measuring cup. Reserve the rest for some other juice. Set aside.

Peel the lemon and cut lengthwise in half. Set aside.

Now, combine mango, cherries, grapes, and lemon in a juicer and process until well juiced. Transfer to serving glasses and stir in the water.

Add few ice cubes and serve immediately.

Nutritional information per serving: Kcal: 302, Protein: 4.8g, Carbs: 86.3g, Fats: 1.7g

27. Grapefruit Apple Juice

Ingredients:

2 large grapefruits, peeled

1 large red apple, cored

2 large strawberries, chopped

1 small ginger knob, peeled

2 oz of coconut water

Preparation:

Peel the grapefruits and divide into wedges. Set aside.

Wash the apple and cut in half. Remove the core and cut into bite-sized pieces. Set aside.

Wash the strawberries and cut into small pieces. Set aside.

Peel the ginger knob and set aside.

Now, combine grapefruits, apple, strawberries, and ginger in a juicer. Process until well juiced and transfer to serving glasses. Stir in the coconut water and refrigerate for 15 minutes, or add some ice before serving.

Nutritional information per serving: Kcal: 302, Protein: 4.8g, Carbs: 86.3g, Fats: 1.7g

28.   Pumpkin Nutmeg Juice

Ingredients:

2 cups of pumpkin, cubed

1 large green apple, cored

1 large cucumber, sliced

1 cup of Swiss chard, torn

2 oz of water

¼ tsp of nutmeg, ground

Preparation:

Peel the pumpkin and cut in half. Scoop out the seeds using a spoon. Cut one large wedge and peel it. Cut into small cubes and fill the measuring cup. Reserve the rest for some other juice.

Wash the apple and cut in half. Remove the core and cut into bite-sized pieces. Set aside.

Wash the cucumber and cut into thin slices. Set aside.

Wash the Swiss chard thoroughly under cold running water. Drain and torn with hands. Set aside.

Now, combine pumpkin, apple, cucumber, and Swiss chards in a juicer. Process until well juiced and stir in the water and nutmeg. Refrigerate for 15 minutes before serving.

Nutritional information per serving: Kcal: 196, Protein: 5.8g, Carbs: 55.4g, Fats: 1.1g

29.   Celery Green Bean Juice

Ingredients:

2 cups of celery, chopped

1 cup of green beans, chopped

1 cup of fresh mint, torn

1 cup of beet greens, torn

1 large cucumber, sliced

2 oz of water

¼ tsp of salt

Preparation:

Wash the celery and cut into small pieces. Set aside.

Wash the green beans and cut into bite-sized pieces. Set aside.

Combine mint and beet greens in a colander. Wash under cold running water and torn with hands. Set aside.

Wash the cucumber and cut into thin slices. Set aside.

Now, combine celery, green beans, mint, beet greens, and cucumber in a juicer. Process until well juiced and transfer to serving glasses. Stir in the water and salt.

Refrigerate for 10 minutes before serving.

Nutritional information per serving: Kcal: 91, Protein: 6.1g, Carbs: 26.1g, Fats: 1g

30.   Strawberry Peach Juice

Ingredients:

1 cup of strawberries, chopped

2 large peaches, pitted

1 large green apple, cored

1 large lemon, peeled

1 large kiwi, peeled

1 large orange, peeled

2 oz of water

Preparation:

Wash the strawberries under cold running water. Remove the green parts and cut into bite-sized pieces. Set aside.

Wash the peaches and cut in half. Remove the pits and cut into small pieces. Set aside.

Wash the apple and cut half. Remove the core and cut into bite-sized pieces. Set aside.

Peel the lemon and kiwi. Cut lengthwise in half and set aside.

Now, combine strawberries, peaches, apple, lemon, and kiwi in a juicer and process until well juiced. Transfer to serving glasses and stir in the water. Add some ice and serve immediately.

Enjoy!

Nutritional information per serving: Kcal: 345, Protein: 7.8g, Carbs: 105g, Fats: 2.3g

31.   Sour Pepper Lemon Juice

Ingredients:

1 large red bell pepper, chopped

1 large lemon, peeled

1 cup of beets, chopped

1 large cucumber, sliced

1 tsp of balsamic vinegar

¼ tsp of salt

2 oz of water

Preparation:

Wash the bell pepper and cut in half. Remove the seeds and chop into small pieces. Set aside.

Peel the lemon and cut lengthwise in half. Set aside.

Wash the beets and trim off the green ends. Cut into bite-sized pieces and fill the measuring cup. Reserve the rest for some other juice. Set aside.

Wash the cucumber and cut into thin slices. Set aside.

Now, combine bell pepper, lemon, beets, and cucumber in a juicer. Process until well juiced and transfer to serving glasses. Stir in the balsamic vinegar, salt, and water.

Refrigerate for 20 minutes before serving.

Nutritional information per serving: Kcal: 130, Protein: 6.4g, Carbs: 39.2g, Fats: 1.2g

32.   Blackberry Apricot Juice

Ingredients:

1 cup of blackberries

1 cup of raspberries

3 large apricots, pitted

1 large red apple, cored

3 large carrots, peeled

Preparation:

Combine blackberries and raspberries in a colander. Wash under cold running water and slightly drain. Set aside.

Wash the apricots and cut in half. Remove the pits and cut into bite-sized pieces. Set aside.

Wash the apple and cut in half. Remove the core and cut into small pieces.

Wash and peel the carrots. Cut into thin slices and set aside.

Now, combine blackberries, raspberries, apricots, apple, and carrots in a juicer. Process until well juiced and transfer to serving glasses. Stir in the water and refrigerate for 20 minutes before serving.

Enjoy!

Nutritional information per serving: Kcal: 301, Protein: 7.6g, Carbs: 97.4g, Fats: 2.9g

33.   Strawberry Avocado Juice

Ingredients:

5 large strawberries, chopped

1 cup of avocado, pitted

1 cup of fresh mint, chopped

1 large apple, cored

1 large lemon, peeled

1 large cucumber, sliced

Preparation:

Wash the strawberries and cut into small pieces. Set aside.

Peel the avocado and cut lengthwise in half. Remove the pit and cut into chunks and fill the measuring cup. Reserve the rest for later.

Wash the mint thoroughly and torn with hands. Set aside.

Wash the apple and cut in half. Remove the core and cut into bite-sized pieces. Set aside.

Peel the lemon and cut lengthwise in half. Set aside.

Wash the cucumber and cut into thin slices. Set aside.

Now, combine strawberries, avocado, mint, lemon, and cucumber in a juicer and process until juiced. Transfer to serving glasses and stir in the water. Add some ice and serve immediately.

Nutritional information per serving: Kcal: 376, Protein: 8.1g, Carbs: 67.8g, Fats: 23.3g

34.   Cantaloupe Carrot Juice

Ingredients:

1 cup of cantaloupe, cubed

3 large carrots, sliced

1 large orange, peeled

1 large green apple, cored

2 oz of coconut water

Preparation:

Cut the cantaloupe in half. Scoop out the seeds and flesh. Cut two wedges and peel them. Chop into cubes and set aside. Reserve the rest of the cantaloupe in a refrigerator.

Wash and peel the carrots. Cut into thin slices and set aside.

Peel the orange and divide into wedges. Set aside.

Wash the apple and cut in half. Remove the core and cut into bite-sized pieces. Set aside.

Now, combine cantaloupe, carrots, orange, and apple in a juicer. Process until well juiced and stir in the coconut water.

Nutritional information per serving: Kcal: 277, Protein: 6g, Carbs: 83g, Fats: 1.4g

35.   Pomegranate Pepper Juice

Ingredients:

1 cup of pomegranate seeds

1 large red bell pepper, chopped

1 cup of cranberries

4 large plums, pitted

1 large green apple, cored

Preparation:

Cut the top of the pomegranate fruit using a sharp knife. Slice down to each of the white membranes inside of the fruit. Pop the seeds into a measuring cup and set aside.

Wash the bell pepper and cut lengthwise in half. Remove the seeds and cut into small pieces. Set aside.

Wash the cranberries thoroughly and drain. Set aside.

Wash the plums and cut in half. Remove the pits and cut into bite-sized pieces. Set aside.

Wash the apple and cut in half. Remove the core and cut into bite-sized pieces. Set aside.

Now, combine pomegranate, cranberries, plums, and apple in a juicer. Process until well juiced and add some ice before serving.

Enjoy!

Nutritional information per serving: Kcal: 277, Protein: 6g, Carbs: 83g, Fats: 1.4g

36.   Zucchini Kiwi Juice

Ingredients:

1 large zucchini, seeded

3 large kiwis, peeled

1 large lime, peeled

1 cup of pomegranate seeds

1 large orange, peeled

Preparation:

Wash the zucchini and cut in half. Scoop out the seeds using a spoon. Cut into small chunks and set aside.

Peel the kiwis and lime. Cut lengthwise in half and set aside.

Cut the top of the pomegranate fruit using a sharp knife. Slice down to each of the white membranes inside of the fruit. Pop the seeds into a measuring cup and set aside.

Peel the orange and divide into wedges. Set aside.

Now, process kiwis, zucchini, lime, pomegranate seeds, and orange in a juicer.

Transfer to a serving glasses and add some ice cubes before serving.

Nutritional information per serving: Kcal: 183, Protein: 8.5g, Carbs: 52.6g, Fats: 1.6g

37.   Blueberry Mango Juice

Ingredients:

1 cup of mango, chopped

1 cup of blueberries

1 large cucumber, sliced

1 large green apple, cored

2 oz of water

Preparation:

Wash the mango and cut into chunks. Fill the measuring cup and reserve the rest for some other juice. Set aside.

Place the blueberries in a colander and wash under cold running water. Drain and set aside.

Wash the apple and remove the core. Cut into bite-sized pieces and set aside.

Now, combine mango, blueberries, and apple in a juicer and process until juiced.

Transfer to serving glasses and stir in the water. Add some ice before serving and enjoy!

Nutritional information per serving: Kcal: 180, Protein: 5.9g, Carbs: 63.5g, Fats: 1.1g

38.   Carrot Lemon Juice

Ingredients:

5 large carrots, sliced

2 large lemons, peeled

1 large green apple, cored

1 cup of Romaine lettuce

2 oz of water

Preparation:

Wash the carrots and cut into thick slices. Set aside.

Peel the lemons and cut lengthwise in half. Set aside.

Wash the apple and remove the core. Cut into bite-sized pieces and set aside.

Wash the lettuce thoroughly under cold running water. Torn with hands and set aside.

Now, process carrots, lettuce, lemon, and apple in a juicer. Transfer to serving glasses and add some ice before serving.

Enjoy!

Nutritional information per serving: Kcal: 232, Protein: 6.1g, Carbs: 74.9g, Fats: 1.7g

39.   Guava Lime Juice

Ingredients:

1 large guava, peeled

1 large lime, peeled

2 large oranges, peeled

1 large cucumber, sliced

2 oz of water

Preparation:

Peel and wash the guava. Cut into small chunks and set aside.

Peel the lime and cut lengthwise in half. Set aside.

Peel the oranges and divide into wedges. Set aside.

Wash the cucumber and cut into thin slices. Set aside.

Now, combine lime, guava, orange, and cucumber in a juicer and process until juiced.

Transfer to serving glasses and stir in the water. Add some ice and serve immediately.

Nutritional information per serving: Kcal: 210, Protein: 7g, Carbs: 65.7g, Fats: 1.3g

40.   Celery Lemon Juice

Ingredients:

1 large lemon, peeled

1 cup of celery, chopped

1 cup of fresh mint, chopped

1 cup of fresh spinach, chopped

2 oz of water

Preparation:

Peel the lemon and cut lengthwise in half. Set aside.

Wash the celery stalks and chop into small pieces. Fill the measuring cup and set aside.

Wash the spinach and mint in a colander. Chop and place in a medium bowl. Set aside.

Now, combine lemon, celery, mint, and spinach in a juicer and process until juiced. Transfer to serving glasses and stir in the water.

Refrigerate for 10 minutes before serving.

Nutritional information per serving: Kcal: 35, Protein: 3.1g, Carbs: 13.2g, Fats: 0.7g

41.   Basil Lemon Juice

Ingredients:

1 cup of fresh basil, chopped

1 large lemon, peeled

1 cup of Swiss chard, chopped

1 large green apple, cored

1 cup of fresh mint, chopped

2 oz of water

Preparation:

Combine basil, Swiss chard, and mint in a large colander. Wash thoroughly under cold running water. Chop into small pieces and set aside.

Peel the lemon and cut lengthwise in half.

Wash the apple and cut in half. Remove the core and cut into bite-sized pieces. Set aside.

Now, combine basil, Swiss chard, mint, lemon, and apple in a juicer and process until well juiced. Transfer to serving glasses and stir in the water.

Refrigerate for 10 minutes before serving.

Enjoy!

Nutritional information per serving: Kcal: 126, Protein: 3.9g, Carbs: 39.1g, Fats: 1.1g

42.   Pineapple Carrot Juice

Ingredients:

1 cup of pineapple chunks

2 large carrots, sliced

1 cup of watercress, torn

1 large lime, peeled

1 small ginger knob, peeled

2 oz of water

Preparation:

Peel the pineapple and cut into small chunks. Set aside.

Wash and peel the carrots. Cut into thin slices and set aside.

Wash the watercress thoroughly under cold running water. Torn with hands and set aside.

Peel the lime and cut lengthwise in half. Set aside.

Peel the ginger root knob and cut into small pieces. Set aside.

Now, combine pineapple, carrots, watercress, lemon, and ginger in a juicer and process until well juiced.

Transfer to serving glasses and stir in water.

Add some ice and serve.

Nutritional information per serving: Kcal: 135, Protein: 3.3g, Carbs: 40.6g, Fats: 3.3g

43. Orange Apple Juice

Ingredients:

3 large oranges, peeled

1 large green apple, cored

1 cup of fresh asparagus, trimmed

¼ tsp of turmeric, ground

2 oz of water

Preparation:

Peel the oranges and divide into wedges. Set aside.

Wash the apple and remove the core. Cut into bite-sized pieces and set aside.

Wash the asparagus thoroughly under cold running water and trim off the woody ends. Cut into small pieces and set aside.

Now, combine oranges, apple, and asparagus in a juicer and process until juiced. Transfer to serving glasses and stir in the turmeric and water.

Refrigerate for 10 minutes before serving.

Nutritional information per serving: Kcal: 316, Protein: 9.1g, Carbs: 98.1g, Fats: 1.2g

44.   Grapefruit Kiwi Juice

Ingredients:

2 large grapefruits, peeled

1 large kiwi, peeled

1 large lime, peeled

2 large celery stalks, chopped

1 cup of red leaf lettuce, chopped

2 oz of water

Preparation:

Peel the grapefruit and divide into wedges. Set aside.

Peel the kiwi and lime. Cut in half and set aside.

Wash and chop the celery stalks into small pieces. Set aside.

Wash the lettuce thoroughly under cold running water and roughly chop it. Set aside.

Now, combine grapefruit, kiwi, celery, and lettuce in a juicer and process until well juiced.

Transfer to serving glasses and stir in the water. Serve immediately.

Nutritional information per serving: Kcal: 233, Protein: 6g, Carbs: 70.7g, Fats: 1.3g

45.   Beet Pear Juice

Ingredients:

2 cups of beets, chopped

1 large pear, cored

1 large red bell pepper, chopped

1 large lemon, peeled

1 small ginger root slice, peeled

3 oz of water

Preparation:

Wash the beets and trim off the green ends. Cut into small pieces and fill the measuring cup. Reserve the greens for some other juice. Set aside.

Wash the pear and cut in half. Remove the core and cut into bite-sized pieces. Set aside.

Wash the bell pepper and cut in half. Remove the seeds and cut into small pieces. Set aside.

Peel the lemon and cut lengthwise in half. Set aside.

Peel the ginger slice and cut in half. Set aside.

Now, combine beets, pear, bell pepper, lemon, and ginger in a juicer. Process until well juiced and transfer to serving glasses.

Stir in the water and add some ice before serving.

Enjoy!

Nutritional information per serving: Kcal: 239, Protein: 7.5g, Carbs: 76.7g, Fats: 1.4g

MEAL RECIPES

1.   Spring Salmon Fillets with Olive Oil Dressing

Ingredients:

1 lb of wild salmon fillets, thinly sliced

2 lbs of wild asparagus

1 tbsp olive oil

1 tsp of sea salt

For the dressing:

1 tbsp of olive oil

1 tbsp of Dijon mustard

2 tbsp of sour cream

1 tsp of fresh parsley, finely chopped

1 tbsp of lemon juice

Preparation:

Preheat the oven to 375°F.

Combine all dressing ingredients in a small mixing bowl. Stir well to combine and set aside.

Cut off the fibrous ends of asparagus and place in a pot of boiling water. Cook until soften and remove from the heat. Drain and set aside.

Place some parchment paper on a large baking sheet. Coat the filets with olive oil and put it in the oven. Bake for 10 minutes or until set. Remove from the heat and transfer to a serving plate. Add asparagus and drizzle with dressing.

Serve.

Nutrition information per serving: Kcal: 272, Protein: 27.4g, Carbs: 9.4g, Fats: 15.7g

2.   Eggs Avocado Salad

Ingredients:

1 medium-sized avocado, chopped

2 large eggs, hard-boiled and chopped

½ cup of cream cheese

1 tsp of lemon juice

1 garlic clove, minced

1 tbsp of fresh parsley, finely chopped

2 tbsp of mayonnaise

¼ tsp of smoked paprika, ground

¼ tsp of salt

Preparation:

Combine cream cheese, lemon juice, mayonnaise, paprika, and salt in a mixing bowl. Whisk well until nicely smooth and set aside.

Combine avocado and hard-boiled eggs in a large salad bowl. Toss to combine and drizzle with marinade. Give it a good stir and refrigerate for 1 hour before using.

Nutrition information per serving: Kcal: 270, Protein: 6.5g, Carbs: 7.5g, Fats: 24.9g

3. Coconut Shrimp Soup

Ingredients:

8 oz of shrimps, peeled and deveined

12 oz of coconut milk

1 cup of corn kernel

4 tbsp of vegetable oil

¼ cup of shallots, thinly sliced

2 tbsp of chives, chopped

1 tsp of vegetable seasoning mix

1 tsp of curry powder

Preparation:

Preheat 2 tablespoons of oil in a large frying skillet over a medium-high temperature. Add shrimps and curry powder and stir well. Cook for about 1-2 minutes, or until slightly browned. Transfer the shrimps to another bowl and reserve the pan. Reduce the temperature to low and add the remaining oil.

Add shallots and chives and cook for about 2-3 minutes. Sprinkle with vegetable seasoning mix and stir well. Add coconut milk, corn kernel, and shrimps and stir again. Cook for 5 minutes and remove from the heat. Garnish with some extra chives and serve.

Nutrition information per serving: Kcal: 425, Protein: 16.5g, Carbs: 14.9g, Fats: 35.4g

4.   Apple Spinach Shake

Ingredients:

1 medium-sized apple, chopped

1 cup of cucumber, peeled and sliced

1 cup of baby spinach, chopped

1 cup of water

1 tbsp of flaxseeds

Preparation:

Combine apple, cucumber and water in a food processor. Blend until nicely smooth and then add all other ingredients. Re-blend for 1 minute and transfer to a serving glasses. Refrigerate for 1 hour before serving, or add few ice cubes and serve immediately.

Nutrition information per serving: Kcal: 88, Protein: 1.7g, Carbs: 18.8g, Fats: 1.4g

5.   Albacore Tuna with Roasted Veggies

Ingredients:

2 cans of Albacore Tuna, minced and drained

4 bell peppers, cut into strips

1 medium-sized onion, sliced

1 cup of tomato sauce

1 small jalapeno pepper, minced

2 large eggs, hard-boiled

¼ cup of anchovies, drained

1 tbsp of lemon juice

3 tbsp of olive oil

¼ tsp of salt

¼ tsp of black pepper, ground

Preparation:

Preheat the oven to 475°F.

Combine lemon juice, oil, salt, and pepper in small mixing bowl. Stir well to combine and set aside to allow flavors to mingle.

Place the peppers and onion on a large greased baking dish. Bake for 20 minutes and add tomato sauce. Cook for another 10 minutes, or until vegetables soften. Remove from the heat and let it cool.

Transfer the vegetables to a large bowl and stir in the jalapeno pepper.

Boil the eggs for about 8-10 minutes over a medium-high temperature. Remove from the heat and drain the water. Place the eggs under the cold water to cool completely. Peel and slice the eggs into wedges. Add the eggs in a salad bowl and toss well to combine with veggies.

Add tuna and give it a good stir. Top with anchovies and sprinkle with extra salt if needed. Enjoy!

Nutrition information per serving: Kcal: 256, Protein: 19.3g, Carbs: 16.1g, Fats: 14.3g

6. Fresh Lime Cucumber Salad

Ingredients:

3.5 oz cucumber, peeled and sliced

1 tbsp of fresh lime juice

3 tbsp of extra virgin olive oil

2 tbsp of parsley, finely chopped

2 garlic cloves, minced

½ tsp of salt

¼ tsp of black pepper, freshly ground

Preparation:

Peel and slice the cucumber. Transfer to a serving platter. Combine the olive oil with fresh lime juice, chopped parsley, crushed garlic cloves, salt, and pepper. Stir well to combine. Pour the mixture over cucumber and let it stand in the refrigerator for about one hour before serving.

Nutrition information per serving: Kcal: 121, Protein: 2.2g, Carbs: 3.1g, Fats: 13.2g

7. Sweet Dijon Chicken

Ingredients:

2 lbs of chicken breasts, skinless and boneless

2 tbsp of Dijon mustard

2 tbsp of raw honey

2 tbsp of red wine vinegar

3 tbsp of lemon juice

2 tbsp of olive oil

¼ tsp of salt

¼ tsp of black pepper, ground

Preparation:

Preheat oven to 350°F.

Combine mustard, honey, vinegar, lemon juice, oil, salt, and pepper in a mixing bowl. Stir well and set aside to allow flavors to mingle.

Place some parchment paper over a baking sheet and spread the chicken filets evenly. Spoon the sauce onto each filet and put it in the oven. Bake for about 1 hour or until, golden brown.

Serve the meat with steamed vegetables or rice. Enjoy.

Nutrition information per serving: Kcal: 355, Protein: 44.1g, Carbs: 6.3g, Fats: 16.1g

8.   Light Fennel Salad with Creamy Yogurt Topping

Ingredients:

7 oz of celery, cut into lengthwise strips

1 small cucumber, cut into lengthwise strips

1 small zucchini, cut into lengthwise strips

1 medium-sized fennel bulb, cut into lengthwise strips

1 tbsp of lemon juice

½ tsp of salt

¼ tsp of black pepper, ground

For the sauce:

10 fl oz of yogurt

3 tbsp of vegetable oil

2 tbsp of lemon juice

½ tsp of salt

¼ tsp of black pepper, ground

1 tsp of dill, finely chopped

Preparation:

Combine all sauce ingredients in a mixing bowl. Stir well and set aside.

Place all vegetables on a serving plate and sprinkle with lemon juice. Season with salt and pepper to taste. Drizzle over the sauce and stir again.

Serve!

Nutritional information per serving: Kcal: 105, Protein: 4.5g, Carbs: 11.6g, Fats: 6.3g

9.   Baked Brussel Sprouts with Garlic and Olive Oil

Ingredients:

1 lb of Brussel sprouts, whole

5 garlic cloves, finely chopped

2 tbsp of olive oil

½ tsp of salt

¼ tsp of black pepper, ground

1 tsp of butter, melted

Preparation:

Preheat the oven to 400°F.

Place the Brussel sprouts in a deep pot. Pour water enough to cover it. Bring it to a boil and reduce the heat. Cook for 10 minutes, or until soften. Remove from the heat and transfer to a large bowl.

Add garlic, olive oil, and melted butter. Season with salt and pepper to taste. Stir well to combine.

Transfer the mixture in a large baking sheet in a single layer. Bake for about 20 minutes. Remove from the heat and serve.

Nutritional information per serving: Kcal: 163, Protein: 3.1g, Carbs: 6.5g, Fats: 13.8g

10. Mint Rice Salad

Ingredients:

1 cup of brown rice, long grain

3 spring onions, finely chopped

½ cup of sweet corn

1 medium-sized red bell pepper

1tsbp of fresh mint, finely chopped

2 tbsp of extra virgin olive oil

1 tbsp of apple cider vinegar

¼ tsp of salt

Preparation:

Place the rice in a deep pot. Add 3 cups of water and bring it to a boil. Reduce the heat, cover and simmer until the water evaporates. Remove from the heat and cool.

Combine the ingredients in a deep bowl. Add olive oil, apple cider vinegar, and some salt to taste. Toss well to combine.

Serve cold.

Nutrition information per serving: Kcal: 395, Protein: 2.4g, Carbs: 37.8g, Fats: 17.7g

11. Broccoli Mushroom Soup with Cheddar

Ingredients:

10 oz of fresh broccoli, chopped

10 of button mushrooms, chopped

2 cups of vegetable broth, unsalted

1 cup of water

¼ cup of skim milk

1 cup of cheddar cheese, crumbled

½ tsp of salt

¼ tsp of black pepper, ground

Preparation:

Place broccoli in a pot of boiling water. Cook until fork-tender and remove from the heat. Drain well and set aside to cool.

Combine mushrooms, vegetable broth, milk, salt, and pepper in a deep pot over a medium-high temperature. Cook until boils, then add broccoli. Reduce the heat to low and cover with a lid. Simmer for 20 minutes. Remove from the heat and let it cool completely. Transfer to a food processor and blend until nicely smooth.

Return the soup to the pot and heat it up. Stir in the cheese. Serve warm.

Nutrition information per serving: Kcal: 115, Protein: 8.9g, Carbs: 5.2g, Fats: 7.0g

12.   Wild Salmon Risotto

Ingredients:

1 lb of wild salmon fillets, skinless and boneless, chopped

2 cups of white rice, long-grain

2 tbsp of maple syrup

1 garlic clove, minced

2 tbsp of olive oil

¼ tsp of salt

¼ tsp of black pepper, ground

Preparation:

Place rice in a large pot. Pour 3 cups of water and bring it to a boil. Cook until water evaporates, or until set. Remove from the heat and set aside to cool.

Preheat the oil in a large skillet over a medium-high temperature. Add maple syrup and garlic. Stir and cook for 1 minute, then add meat chops. Sprinkle with salt and pepper and cook until golden brown, stirring occasionally.

Nutrition information per serving: Kcal: 575, Protein: 28.7g, Carbs: 81.0g, Fats: 14.6g

13.   Stewed Spinach with Fresh Coriander

Ingredients:

7oz fresh spinach, chopped

2 tbsp fresh coriander, finely chopped

1 tsp of apple cider vinegar

3 tbsp extra-virgin olive oil

Freshwater

Preparation:

Fill in a large saucepan with fresh water and bring to a boil. Wash the spinach and add to the saucepan. Cover and reduce the heat to minimum. Cook for about 2-3 minutes, until spinach has wilted.

Remove from the heat and drain. Allow it to cool for a while.

Transfer the spinach to a skillet. Add olive oil and stir-fry for several minutes, stirring constantly. Remove from the heat and season with fresh coriander and apple cider vinegar. Serve.

Nutrition information per serving: Kcal: 38, Protein: 3.0g, Carbs: 5.4g, Fats: 7.3g

14.   Creamy Apple and Turkey Pitas

Ingredients:

8 oz of turkey breasts, skinless and boneless

1 medium-sized apple, cored and sliced

1 small onion, sliced

2 medium-sized bell pepper, striped

½ cup of plain yogurt

1 garlic clove, minced

2 tbsp of olive oil

2 tbsp of lemon juice

¼ tsp of dried mint, ground

3 pita breads, whole-wheat, halved

Preparation:

Combine apple slices with lemon juice in a medium bowl. Set aside to allow juice to penetrate into an apple.

Preheat the oil in a large nonstick skillet over a medium-high temperature. Add onion, pepper and cook until peppers soften. Add meat and stir well. Cook for about 10-

15 minutes, or until set. Reduce the heat to low and stir in the apple mixture. Cook for 2 minutes more, stirring constantly. Remove from the heat.

Combine yogurt, garlic, and mint. Give it a good stir and set aside.

Fold the pitas in half and spoon the meat mixture. Add 1 tablespoon of yogurt mixture and serve.

Nutrition information per serving: Kcal: 215, Protein: 11.1g, Carbs: 29.2g, Fats: 6.1g

15.   Sweet Carrot Salad

Ingredients:

1 medium-sized carrot, sliced

2oz baby spinach, chopped

1 medium-sized tomato, finely chopped

2 oz of rice spaghetti, soaked

¼ cup of fresh blueberries

For the dressing:

¼ cup of honey

¼ cup of fresh lime juice

1 tsp of Dijon mustard

¼ tbsp of cumin, ground

Preparation:

Soak the rice spaghetti in water for about 15 minutes. Drain and transfer to a bowl. Set aside.

Add chopped spinach, tomato, carrot, and blueberries. Toss to combine.

In another bowl, combine the marinade ingredients and mix well. Drizzle over the salad. Serve.

Nutrition information per serving: Kcal: 98 Protein: 4.5g, Carbs: 19.2g, Fats: 6.3g

16.   Poached Salmon

Ingredients:

1 lb of wild salmon filets, sliced

2 tbsp of lemon juice

1 large onion, sliced

1 large carrot, sliced

1 tsp of fresh dill, finely chopped

4 cups of water

1-2 bay leaves

Preparation:

Combine lemon juice, onion, carrot, and dill in a large saucepan. Pour 4 cups of water and stir well. Bring it to a boil and then reduce the heat to low. Simmer for about 5-6 minutes. Transfer the mixture to a large bowl and reserve the saucepan.

Add salmon filets and spread on the bottom of the pan. Now, return the mixture to the pan. Cover with a lid and cook for about 20-25 minutes, or until meat flakes.

Nutrition information per serving: Kcal: 238, Protein: 24.2g, Carbs: 7.2g, Fats: 12.4g

17.   Spring Onions Chicken

Ingredients:

2 lbs of chicken breasts, skinless and boneless

¼ cup of all-purpose flour

½ tsp of Cayenne pepper, ground

¼ tsp of black pepper, ground

¼ tsp of salt

For the sauce:

1 cup of chicken broth, unsalted

2 large red bell peppers, finely chopped

1 tbsp of olive oil

2 tsp of all-purpose flour

1 tsp of Cayenne pepper, ground

1 cup of spring onions, finely chopped

2 tbsp of apple cider vinegar

¼ tsp of salt

Preparation:

Preheat oven to 375°F.

Preheat the oil in a large saucepan over a medium-high temperature. Add bell peppers and spring onions. Cook until soften. Add chicken broth and sprinkle with cayenne pepper. Stir well and cook for about 2-3 minutes more. Remove from the heat and add vinegar and salt. Give it a good stir and set aside to cool.

Combine flour, cayenne pepper, pepper, and salt in a large bowl. Add the meat and toss well to combine. Set aside for 15 minutes to allow flavors to penetrate to meat. Transfer the meat to a large greased baking sheet and put it in the oven. Bake for 20 minutes or until golden brown. Add the sauce and bake for another 15 minutes. Remove from the heat and let it cool for a while.

Serve.

Nutrition information per serving: Kcal: 357, Protein: 46.0g, Carbs: 9.4g, Fats: 13.9g

18.   Green Potato Omelet

Ingredients:

6 free-range eggs

3 small potatoes, peeled and sliced

1 cup of spring onions, finely chopped

1 tbsp of skim milk

1 tbsp of olive oil

¼ tsp of salt

1 tsp of vegetable seasoning mix

¼ tsp of black pepper, ground

Preparation:

Place the potatoes in a pot of boiling water. Cook until fork-tender. Remove from the heat and drain. Set aside.

Whisk the eggs, milk, salt, and pepper in a mixing bowl. Set aside.

Preheat the oil in a large nonstick frying pan and add spring onions. Cook 1 minute, then add potatoes. Add the egg mixture and cook until eggs are set. Sprinkle with vegetable seasoning mix and remove from the heat. Fold the omelet and serve immediately.

Nutrition information per serving: Kcal: 222, Protein: 11.1g, Carbs: 22.7g, Fats: 10.2g

19.   Blueberry Spinach Quinoa Smoothie

Ingredients:

1 cup of fresh blueberries

1 cup of white quinoa, pre-cooked

1 cup of fresh spinach, roughly chopped

1 cup of plain yogurt

1 cup of skim milk

1 tbsp of honey

1 tsp of chia seeds

2 mint leaves

Preparation:

Place quinoa in a large pot. Add 3 cups of water and cook until set. Remove from the heat and fluff with a fork. Drain and set aside to cool for a while.

Combine blueberries, spinach, yogurt, milk, honey, and quinoa in a food processor. Blend until nicely smooth. Top with chia seeds and garnish with mint leaves. Refrigerate 1 hour before serving.

Nutrition information per serving: Kcal: 261, Protein: 12.0g, Carbs: 44.4g, Fats: 3.5g

20. Cranberry Rice Balls

Ingredients:

1 cup of brown rice, pre-cooked

1 cup of dried cranberries

½ cup of cornstarch

5 tbsp of orange juice

2 tbsp of lemon juice

1 tsp of cumin, ground

2 large eggs

2 tbsp of olive oil

¼ tsp of salt

¼ tsp of black pepper, ground

1 tbsp of fresh parsley, finely chopped

Preparation:

Place rice in a deep pot and add 3 cups of water. Bring it to a boil and cook until set. Remove from the heat and let it cool completely.

Combine rice, cranberries, eggs, salt, and pepper. Stir well to combine. Shape the balls and roll them in cornstarch.

Preheat the oil in a large pot over a medium-high temperature. Add balls and cook for about 4-5 minutes, or until browned.

Meanwhile, combine orange juice, lemon juice, cumin, salt, and pepper. Add 1 cup of water and cover with a lid. Reduce the heat to low and cook for about 3-4 hours. Remove from the heat and sprinkle with parsley for extra taste.

Nutrition information per serving: Kcal: 476, Protein: 9.4g, Carbs: 74.7g, Fats: 14.7g

21.   Cabbage Salad with Pecans

Ingredients:

1 large red cabbage head, shredded

1 cup of pecans, roughly chopped

1 cup of spring onions, finely chopped

½ cup of Feta cheese, crumbled

4 tbsp of balsamic vinegar

4 tbsp of olive oil

1 tbsp of milk

¼ tsp of salt

¼ tsp of black pepper, ground

Preparation:

Combine vinegar, oil, milk, salt, and pepper in a mixing bowl. Set aside to allow flavors to meld.

Combine cabbage, pecans, and spring onions in a large salad bowl. Toss well to combine. Top with cheese and drizzle with previously made dressing.

Serve immediately.

Nutrition information per serving: Kcal: 252, Protein: 5.9g, Carbs: 13.9g, Fats: 20.8g

22.   Apricot Chicken Burgers

Ingredients:

12 oz of chicken breasts, pre-cooked, shredded

2 cups of apricots, chopped

1 medium-sized onion, sliced

3 tbsp of yellow mustard

1 tbsp of apple cider vinegar

2 garlic cloves, crushed

½ tsp of salt

½ tsp of black pepper, ground

2 lettuce leaves

2 burger buns, multigrain

Preparation:

Combine meat, apricots, onion, mustard, vinegar, garlic, salt, and pepper in a slow cooker. Pour enough water to cover all ingredients. Seal the lid and cook for about 6-7 hours. Remove from the heat and let it cool completely.

Place a lettuce leaf on a burger bun and spoon the meat mixture onto it. Secure with a toothpick. If you like, you can heat the burgers in a microwave.

Serve.

Nutrition information per serving: Kcal: 443, Protein: 53.1g, Carbs: 34.9g, Fats: 14.6g

23.   Black Bean Soup

Ingredients:

2 cans of black beans

2 cups of vegetable broth, unsalted

1 medium-sized onion, finely chopped

1 small red onion, finely chopped

1 garlic clove, minced

1 tbsp of cilantro, finely chopped

3 tbsp of olive oil

1 tsp of cumin, ground

½ tsp of salt

¼ tsp of black pepper, ground

Preparation:

Preheat the oil in a large nonstick skillet over a medium-high temperature. Add onion and red onion and stir-fry until translucent. Sprinkle with cumin and add garlic. Cook for 1 minute more, stirring constantly.

Add 1 can of beans and vegetable broth. Reduce the heat to low, cover with a lid and simmer until beans slightly soften. Remove from the heat and transfer the mixture to a food processor. Blend until smooth and return to the skillet.

Stir in the remaining beans and cook for 1 hour on low temperature. Just before set, add cilantro, salt, and pepper and give it a good stir. Remove from the heat and serve warm.

Nutrition information per serving: Kcal: 461, Protein: 24.0g, Carbs: 65.4g, Fats: 12.7g

24. Casserole di Italia

Ingredients:

1 lb of button mushrooms, sliced

1 medium-sized eggplant, sliced

2 medium-sized bell pepper, sliced

1 small onion, sliced

1 small zucchini, sliced

3 tbsp of olive oil

3 cups of tomato sauce, unsalted

4 oz of Mozzarella cheese, shredded

½ tsp of salt

Preparation:

Preheat the oven to 375°F.

Combine vegetables in a large bowl. Add 2 tablespoons of olive oil and stir to coat well. Transfer to a large nonstick saucepan over a medium-high temperature. Sprinkle with salt and cook until fork-tender. Remove from the heat.

Use the remaining oil to grease a large baking dish. Spread the tomato sauce on the bottom. Add vegetables and spread in one layer. Add another layer of tomato sauce and sprinkle with cheese. Put it in the oven and bake for about 25-30 minutes, or until set.

Nutrition information per serving: Kcal: 200, Protein: 10.8g, Carbs: 19.4g, Fats: 11.1g

25.   Sweet Orange Potatoes with Thyme

Ingredients:

3 cups of sweet potatoes, peeled and cut into bite-sized pieces

2 medium-sized onions, chopped

3 tbsp of olive oil

2 oz of orange juice

½ tsp of dried thyme, ground

½ tsp of salt

¼ tsp of black pepper, ground

2 tbsp of almonds, roughly chopped

Preparation:

Preheat the oven to 400°F.

Combine orange juice, olive oil, thyme, salt, and pepper in a mixing bowl. Stir well to combine and set aside.

Grease a large baking dish with oil. Place potatoes and onions and spread evenly in one layer. Pour in previously made sauce and cover with a lid or piece of aluminum foil.

Put it in the oven and bake for about 30 minutes, or until set.

Remove from the oven and top with almonds. Serve.

Nutrition information per serving: Kcal: 269, Protein: 3.1g, Carbs: 38.8g, Fats: 12.3g

26. Grapefruit Pomegranate Smoothie

Ingredients:

1 medium-sized grapefruit, peeled and wedged

1 cup of plain yogurt

2 oz of pomegranate juice

1 tbsp of honey

2 tbsp of cashews

1 tbsp of pomegranate seeds

Preparation:

Combine grapefruit, yogurt, juice, honey, and cashews in a food processor. Blend until nicely smooth. Transfer to a serving glasses. Refrigerate for 1 hour and top with pomegranate seeds before serving.

Nutrition information per serving: Kcal: 228, Protein: 9.1g, Carbs: 35.0g, Fats: 5.6g

27. Peanut Butter Chicken Wings

Ingredients:

6 chicken wings

3 tbsp of peanut butter

½ tsp of salt

1 tbsp of vegetable oil

1 tsp of fresh ginger, grated

1 cup of water

Preparation:

Combine peanut butter, oil, ginger, salt, water in mixing bowl. Stir well to combine and set aside.

Place chicken wings in a slow cooker or a deep pot. Pour the peanut butter mixture and seal the lid. Cook for about 5-6 hours, or until set.

Remove from the heat and serve with rice or steamed vegetables. However, this is optional.

Nutrition information per serving: Kcal: 421, Protein: 47.4g, Carbs: 3.6g, Fats: 23.7g

28.   Apple Quinoa Salad

Ingredients:

1 large apple, cored and grated

2 cups of white quinoa, pre-cooked

2 medium-sized carrots, grated

1 cup of spring onions, finely chopped

3 tbsp of flaxseed oil

2 tbsp of balsamic vinegar

2 tsp of maple syrup

¼ tsp of salt

Preparation:

Place quinoa in a medium pot. Pour water enough to cover ingredients and cook until set, or until water evaporates. Set aside to cool.

Meanwhile, combine maple syrup, flaxseed oil, salt, and balsamic vinegar in a mixing bowl. Stir well and set aside to allow flavors to meld.

Combine, apple, carrots, onions, and quinoa in a large salad bowl. Drizzle with dressing and refrigerate for 20 minutes before serving.

Nutrition information per serving: Kcal: 470, Protein: 12.9g, Carbs: 69.4g, Fats: 15.8g

29.   Tuna Balsamico

Ingredients:

1 lb of fresh tuna filets

1 medium-sized onion, sliced

2 garlic cloves, minced

2 tbsp of olive oil

2 tbsp of fresh parsley, finely chopped

1 shallot, minced

1 cup of balsamic vinegar

½ tsp of salt

¼ tsp of black pepper, ground

Preparation:

Preheat the broiler to medium-high temperature.

Combine shallot, garlic, vinegar, salt, and honey in a mixing bowl. Set aside.

Preheat 1 tablespoon of oil in a large skillet over a medium-high temperature. Add the onions and stir-fry until translucent. Reduce the temperature to low and add vinegar mixture. Stir well and cook for 1 minute. Remove from the heat and set aside.

Preheat the remaining oil in the same skillet over a medium-high temperature. Add filets and sprinkle with some salt and pepper to taste. Broil for about 4-5 minutes on each side, or until set. Remove from the heat and drizzle with prepared vinegar dressing.

Serve warm.

Nutrition information per serving: Kcal: 298, Protein: 30.6g, Carbs: 3.8g, Fats: 16.2g

30.   Taco Stew

Ingredients:

1 lb of lean beef, ground

1 large red onion, chopped

1 can of tomatoes, diced

1 can of kidney beans

1 can of corn

1 cup of water

1 tsp of taco seasoning mix

1 tsp of chili pepper, ground

2 tbsp of cheddar cheese, shredded

Preparation:

Combine all ingredients in a slow cooker. Cook on high temperature until boils, then reduce to low and cook for 1 hours.

Remove from the heat and garnish with cheese. Serve warm.

Nutrition information per serving: Kcal: 292, Protein: 31.8g, Carbs: 27.5g, Fats: 6.2g

31.   Cherry Vanilla Pancakes

Ingredients

½ cup of almond flour

1 free-range egg

½ tsp of baking powder

¼ tsp of salt

2 tbsp of sour cream

1 tbsp of vanilla extract

2 tbsp of oil (for frying)

2 tbsp of almonds, chopped

2 tbsp of cherry jam

Preparation:

Combine flour, baking powder, and salt in a mixing bowl. In a separate bowl, whisk the eggs, vanilla extract, and sour cream. Combine these two mixtures and stir well until you get nice batter.

Preheat 1 tablespoon of oil in a nonstick pan over a medium-high temperature. Spoon about 2-3 tablespoons of mixture and cook until crisp and browned on each side.

Remove from the heat and spread the cherry jam and roll or fold pancakes. Serve with ice cream, whipped cream, or liquid chocolate.

Nutrition information per serving: Kcal: 423, Protein: 8.6g, Carbs: 47.7g, Fats: 21.7g

32.   Veal Steaks with Green Beans

Ingredients:

2 lbs of veal steaks, thinly sliced

2 cups of green beans, pre-cooked

¼ cup of white wine vinegar

2 tbsp of olive oil

1 cup of chicken stock, unsalted

1 tbsp of yellow mustard

1 tbsp of butter, melted

1 tbsp of lemon juice

1 tbsp of fresh parsley, finely chopped

Preparation:

Place green beans in a pot of boiling water. Sprinkle with a pinch of salt and cook until soften. Remove from the heat and drain well. Set aside.

Combine vinegar, mustard, butter, lemon juice, and parsley in a mixing bowl. Stir well to combine and set aside to allow flavors to meld.

Preheat oil in a large nonstick skillet over a medium-high temperature. Add steaks and cook on both sides until crisp and browned. Add chicken stock and water. Cook until reduced and set.

Remove from the heat and serve with green beans. Drizzle with marinade before serving.

Nutrition information per serving: Kcal: 339, Protein: 40.7g, Carbs: 3.0g, Fats: 17.3g

33.   Orzo Vegetable Salad

Ingredients:

1 cup of orzo pasta, pre-cooked

3 large bell peppers, chopped

1 medium-sized red onion, chopped

2 tbsp of fresh parsley, finely chopped

1 medium-sized carrot, chopped

1 garlic clove, minced

3 tbsp of extra-virgin olive oil

2 tbsp of lemon juice

¼ tsp of lime zest

¼ tsp of black pepper, ground

½ tsp of salt

Preparation:

Combine lemon juice, garlic, salt, pepper, oil, and lime zest in a mixing bowl. Stir all well set aside to allow flavors to meld.

Use package instructions to cook orzo pasta, or put it in a pot of boiling water and cook for about 10-12 minutes, or until soften. Drain well and set aside to cool completely.

Now, transfer the pasta to the salad bowl. Stir in peppers, onion, parsley, and carrots. Drizzle with dressing and serve immediately.

Nutrition information per serving: Kcal: 248, Protein: 5.7g, Carbs: 32.0g, Fats: 11.7g

34. Choco-Cherry Smoothie

Ingredients:

1 cup of frozen cherries

¼ cup of frozen strawberries

1 cup of Greek yogurt

1 tbsp of honey

1 tsp of cocoa powder

1 tbsp of chocolate chips

1 tbsp of chia seeds

Preparation:

Combine all ingredients in a food processor except chia seeds. Blend until nicely smooth. Transfer to a serving glasses. Top with chia seeds and refrigerate or add few ice cubes before serving.

Nutrition information per serving: Kcal: 181, Protein: 13.4g, Carbs: 27.5g, Fats: 4.8g

35. Salmon Croquettes with Cucumber

Ingredients:

1 lb of fresh salmon fillets, skinless and boneless, chopped

1 large cucumber, sliced

1 small red onion, finely chopped

1 small bell pepper, finely chopped

2 bread slices, mixed grain

½ cup of breadcrumbs

5 tbsp of mayonnaise

1 tbsp of fresh parsley, finely chopped

½ tsp of salt

¼ tsp of black pepper, ground

Preparation:

Preheat the oven to 375°F.

Combine meat, onion, pepper, bread, parsley, and mayonnaise in a large bowl. Sprinkle with some salt and pepper to taste and stir well to combine.

Shape the croquettes and roll them in breadcrumbs. Spread over a large greased baking sheet. Put it in the oven and bake for about 25-30 minutes, or until nicely crisp. Remove from the heat and serve with cucumber slices.

Nutrition information per serving: Kcal: 315, Protein: 25.3g, Carbs: 23.1g, Fats: 14.2g

36. Hot Tomato Soup

Ingredients:

1 lb of tomatoes, diced

1 cup of tomato sauce

1 small onion, finely chopped

2 garlic cloves, minced

2 tbsp of olive oil

1 cup of vegetable stock, unsalted

½ cup of fresh chives, finely chopped

1 tsp of chili pepper, ground

¼ tsp of black pepper, ground

½ tsp of salt

½ tsp of dried oregano, ground

1 bread slice, chopped

2 bay leaves

Preparation:

Place tomatoes in a food processor and blend until smooth. Set aside.

Preheat the oil in deep pot over a medium-high temperature. Add onions, garlic, and bay leaves. Stir-fry until translucent.

Add pureed tomatoes and tomato sauce and cook for about 4-5 minutes, stirring constantly. Add bread slices and sprinkle with salt and pepper to taste. Stir once and vegetable stock and chili pepper. Add water to adjust the thickness of the soup. Cook for 10 minutes and reduce the heat to low. Cook until for about 45 minutes, or until set. Remove from the heat and stir in chives. Sprinkle with oregano for some extra taste.

Serve warm.

Nutrition information per serving: Kcal: 114, Protein: 2.5g, Carbs: 11.6g, Fats: 7.5g

37.   Chicken Pasta with Veggies

Ingredients:

1 lb of chicken breasts, pre-cooked, cubed

8 oz of spaghetti pasta, pre-cooked

1 large tomato, diced

1 cup of button mushrooms, chopped

1 small zucchini, sliced

1 cup of skim milk

2 tbsp of Parmesan cheese, grated

2 tbsp of olive oil

1 garlic clove, minced

¼ tsp of chili pepper, ground

1 tsp of dried basil, ground

¼ tsp of black pepper, ground

½ tsp of salt

Preparation:

Cook pasta using package instructions. Drain well and set aside.

Preheat the oil in a large skillet over a medium-high temperature. Add garlic, basil, vegetables, and mushrooms. Stir well and cook for about 4-5 minutes, or until soften. Add pasta and toss to combine. Cook for another 2-3 minutes.

Now, add meat, milk and cook until all heated through. Reduce the heat to low, add tomato, chili, cheese, and 1 cup of water. Cover with a lid and cook for 20 minutes, or until set. Stir well and add some extra salt and pepper to taste, if needed.

Serve warm.

Nutrition information per serving: Kcal: 320, Protein: 28.4g, Carbs: 25.2g, Fats: 11.3g

38.   Tomato Couscous

Ingredients:

1 cup of couscous

2 large tomatoes, diced

½ cup of Mozzarella cheese

¼ cup of fresh basil, finely chopped

1 garlic clove, minced

4 tbsp of shallots, minced

1 tsp of balsamic vinegar

3 tbsp of olive oil

½ tsp of salt

¼ tsp of black pepper, ground

1 cup of water

Preparation:

Combine cheese, vinegar, oil, garlic, tomato, shallots, salt, and pepper in a medium bowl. Stir well and cover with a lid or foil. Refrigerate for 30 minutes to allow flavors to meld.

Pour water in a deep pot and bring it to a boil. Gently stir in couscous. Remove from the heat and fluff with a fork. Set aside to cool for a while.

Now, combine cooked couscous and tomato mixture in a large bowl. Sprinkle with basil and serve.

Nutrition information per serving: Kcal: 288, Protein: 7.7g, Carbs: 39.2g, Fats: 11.6g

39.   Kefir Cheese Omelet

Ingredients:

¼ cup of fresh goat's cheese

¼ cup of kefir cheese, crumbled

2 tbsp of Feta cheese, crumbled

¼ cup of milk

2 large eggs

¼ tsp of salt

1 tbsp of olive oil

Preparation:

Heat up some olive oil in a large skillet over a medium-high temperature. Combine the cheese and stir-fry for several minutes. Add milk and cook until cheese melts.

Crack two eggs, add some salt to taste and mix with a fork. Cook until eggs are set. Serve warm.

Nutrition information per serving: Kcal: 337, Protein: 16.1g, Carbs: 4.4g, Fats: 30.7g

40.   Meatballs with Onions and Rosemary

Ingredients:

1 lb of minced meat (70% beef brisket and 30% lamb shoulder)

1 large onion, peeled and finely chopped

1 tbsp of finely chopped, fresh rosemary

1 large egg

½ tsp of salt

¼ tsp of black pepper, ground

2 tbsp of all-purpose flour

1 tbsp of olive oil

Preparation:

Combine the ingredients in a large bowl. Add about two tablespoons of oil in the mixture and shape the meatballs using your hands.

Heat up some oil in a large skillet, over a medium-high temperature. Fry the meatballs for about 10 minutes, or until lightly charred. Remove from the heat and serve.

Nutrition information per serving: Kcal: 291, Protein: 36.8g, Carbs: 7.2g, Fats: 12.0g

41.   Orange Arugula Salad with Lentils

Ingredients:

½ cup of cooked lentils,

½ cup of finely chopped arugula

½ cucumber, sliced

½ orange, peeled and sectioned

½ carrot, sliced

½ green bell pepper, sliced

¼ cup of fresh cranberries

Balsamic vinaigrette:

¼ cup of olive oil

½ tsp of ground red pepper

¼ tsp of salt

1 tsp of balsamic vinegar

Preparation:

Combine all vegetables in a large bowl. Add lentils and mix well. Set aside.

In a smaller bowl, whisk balsamic vinegar, olive oil, salt, and red pepper. Pour the vinaigrette over the vegetables and mix well. Top with orange and cranberries. Serve cold.

Nutrition information per serving: Kcal: 222, Protein: 7.0g, Carbs: 21.2g, Fats: 13.0g

42. Chicken Salad with Spinach

Ingredients:

1 piece of chicken breast, 0.5 inch thick, boneless and skinless

1 cup of finely chopped lettuce

½ cup of beans, pre-cooked

1 tbsp of fresh lime juice

1 tbsp of vegetable oil

¼ tsp of salt

¼ tsp of spinach, chopped

Preparation:

Preheat a non-stick grill pan over a medium-high temperature. Wash and pat dry the meat using a kitchen paper. Grill for about 4-5 minutes on each side. You can use some water if necessary. Several tablespoons at a time will be enough to make the process easier. Remove from the heat and cut into several pieces.

Combine the meat with other ingredients, toss with vegetable oil, fresh lime juice, and a pinch of salt. Serve.

Nutrition information per serving: Kcal: 319, Protein: 26.4g, Carbs: 8.0g, Fats: 20.4g

43.   Breakfast Casserole

Ingredients:

1 lb of spinach, finely chopped

8 oz of cherry tomatoes

5 large eggs

½ cup of all-purpose flour

2 cups of skim milk

1 cup of goat's cheese

1 tbsp of dried oregano, ground

½ tsp of salt

¼ tsp of black pepper, ground

Preparation:

Preheat the oven to 400°F.

Line some baking paper over a small casserole dish. Set aside.

Briefly, boil the spinach. Remove from the heat and drain. Place in a casserole dish.

In a medium-sized bowl, combine the cheese, milk, eggs, flour, oregano, salt, and pepper. Whisk together with an electric mixer. Add cherry tomatoes and pour this mixture over spinach.

Bake for about 20 minutes. Remove from the oven and let it cool. Serve.

Nutrition information per serving: Kcal: 192, Protein: 14.1g, Carbs: 17.2g, Fats: 7.6g

44.   Grilled Trout with Rosemary and Mint

Ingredients:

2 lbs of fresh trout, cleaned, boneless

½ cup of olive oil

1 medium-sized lemon, sliced

1 tbsp of dry mint, ground

3 garlic cloves, crushed

¼ tsp of red pepper, ground

½ tsp of salt

Several rosemary sprigs

Preparation:

Preheat the grill to a high temperature.

Combine the olive oil, dry mint, crushed garlic cloves, and red pepper in mixing bowl. Stir well and set aside to allow flavors to meld.

Wash and clean the fish. Cut lengthwise and remove entrails.

Brush the fish with marinade and stuff with lemon slices and rosemary sprigs.

Grill for about 5-7 minutes on each side. Remove from the heat and serve with steamed spinach or cooked potatoes. This is, however, optional.

Nutrition information per serving: Kcal: 436, Protein: 40.4g, Carbs: 1.1g, Fats: 29.6g

45.   Creamy Greek Pita

Ingredients:

2 lbs of all-purpose flour

2 tbsp of dry yeast

1 tbsp of liquid honey

1 tsp of salt

3 ½ cups of water

1 tbsp of black cumin, ground

Preparation:

Preheat the oven to 400°F.

Whisk together dry yeast, honey, salt, and about ¼ cup of warm water. Allow it to stand for about 20 minutes.

Combine the all-purpose flour with the yeast mixture and some water (enough to create a smooth dough). Cover with a cotton cloth and keep it in a warm place for about 40 minutes.

Shape 8 equal bowl and gently press with your hands. Sprinkle with black cumin and bake for 10 minutes.

For the chicken filling:

8 oz of chicken breasts, boneless and skinless

1 medium-sized onion, peeled and finely chopped

5 tbsp of olive oil

1 tbsp of homemade tomato paste

1 tsp of fresh thyme, finely chopped

1 tsp of black cumin

½ tsp of salt

¼ tsp of black pepper, ground

Preparation:

Wash and cut the meat into long, thin strips. Combine the other ingredients in a bowl. Place the meat in it and cover with foil. Allow it to stand for about an hour.

Preheat a non-stick, grill pan over a medium-high temperature. Fry the chicken (with the marinade) for about 10-15 minutes. Stir constantly.

Use this mixture to fill each pita.

Yogurt topping:

Ingredients:

1 cup of Greek yogurt

1 garlic clove

1 tbsp of olive oil

¼ tsp of salt

Preparation:

Combine the ingredients in a bowl. Keep in the refrigerator and top each pita with this mixture.

Nutrition information per serving: Kcal: 534, Protein: 19.4g, Carbs: 90.2g, Fats: 12.4g

46.   Grill Platter

Ingredients:

3 oz of tomatoes, sliced

3 oz of red bell peppers, halved

3 oz of yellow bell peppers, halved

3 oz of onions, sliced

3 oz of eggplant, peeled and sliced

For the marinade:

2 cups of olive oil

5 garlic cloves

1 cup of fresh parsley, finely chopped

¼ cup of fresh thyme, chopped

½ tsp of salt

¼ tsp of black pepper, ground

Preparation:

Combine the marinade ingredients in a large bowl. Wash and cut the vegetables and place in the marinade. Let it stand for 20 minutes.

Preheat an electric grill over a medium-high temperature. Grill for several minutes. Remove from the grill and serve.

Nutrition information per serving: Kcal: 639, Protein: 2.3g, Carbs: 14.5g, Fats: 67.8g

47.   Grilled Smelts

Ingredients:

1 lb of fresh smelts

1 cup of olive oil

½ lemon, sliced

¼ cup of lemon juice

1 tsp of dry rosemary, ground

1 tbsp of fresh parsley, finely chopped

3 garlic cloves, crushed

¼ tsp of sea salt

Preparation:

Wash and drain the fish.

Combine the olive oil, lemon juice, dry rosemary, fresh parsley, crushed garlic cloves, and sea salt in a large bowl. Soak the fish in this marinade and leave in the refrigerator for at least 30 minutes (it can stand in the refrigerator up to 2 hours).

Meanwhile, preheat a grill pan over a medium-high temperature.

Remove the fish from the refrigerator and grill for about 10 minutes. Add some of the marinade while grilling (one or two tablespoons at a time).

Nutrition information per serving: Kcal: 581, Protein: 25.9g, Carbs: 1.3g, Fats: 54.1g

48.   Homemade Sweet Tomato Paste

Ingredients:

2 lbs of fresh tomatoes

1 cup of white wine

1 medium-sized onion, peeled and finely chopped

4 garlic cloves, crushed

2 basil leaves

A handful of chopped parsley

1 tsp of freshly ground red pepper

1 tsp of dry oregano

2 tbsp of sugar

1 tbsp of olive oil

Preparation:

Preheat the olive oil over a medium-high temperature. Add chopped onion and garlic. Stir-fry for several minutes, stirring constantly.

Peel and roughly chop the tomatoes. Place in the skillet and reduce the heat to low. Add the remaining ingredients and cook until the tomatoes soften, for about 40 minutes. Add some water when necessary.

Spread the mixture over a toast and serve with beans, cheese, or olives.

Nutrition information per serving: Kcal: 581, Protein: 25.9g, Carbs: 1.3g, Fats: 54.1g

49. Swiss Chard with Potatoes

Ingredients:

1 lb of Swiss chard

1 medium-sized potato, chopped

½ cup of olive oil

¼ tsp of salt

Water

Preparation:

Rinse the Swiss chard and transfer to a deep pot. Add enough water to cover and briefly boil (for about five minutes). Remove from the heat and drain. Set aside.

Peel and chop the potato into small cubes. Pour the olive oil in a deep, large pot, and add about 1 cup of water. Place the potato in it and cook until soft. This should take about 15 minutes. Now add the Swiss chard, mix well and cook for 10 more minutes. Serve.

Nutrition information per serving: Kcal: 279, Protein: 3.1g, Carbs: 13.5g, Fats: 25.6g

50.   Italian Seafood and Bell Pepper Salad

Ingredients:

1 small cucumber sliced

½ red bell pepper, sliced

1 cup of fresh seafood mix

1 onion, peeled and finely chopped

3 garlic cloves, crushed

¼ cup of fresh orange juice

5 tbsp of extra virgin olive oil

Fresh lettuce leaves, rinsed

¼ tsp of salt

Preparation:

In a large skillet, heat up 3 tablespoons of extra virgin olive oil over a medium-high temperature. Add chopped onion and crushed garlic. Stir-fry for about 5 minutes. Reduce the heat to minimum and add 1 cup of frozen seafood mix. Cover and cook for about 15 minutes, until soft. Remove from the heat and allow it to cool for a while.

Meanwhile, combine the vegetables in a bowl. Add the remaining 2 tablespoons of olive oil, fresh orange juice and a little salt. Toss well to combine.

Top with seafood mix and serve immediately.

Nutrition information per serving: Kcal: 230, Protein: 5.4g, Carbs: 13.7g, Fats: 18.7g

51. Spring Turkey Breast

Ingredients:

2 lbs of turkey breasts, boneless and skinless

1 cup of olive oil

4 cloves of garlic

2 tbsp apple cider vinegar

5 tbsp fresh parsley, finely chopped

1 tsp dry oregano, ground

½ tsp salt

Preparation:

Wash and pat dry the meat. Set aside.

Combine all the other ingredients in a large bowl. Place the meat in it and marinate for about an hour.

Preheat the grill pan and grill the meat for about 10 minutes on each side. You can add some marinade while frying (1 tablespoon will be enough).

You can serve it with boiled potato and broccoli. Peel the potato and slice into thin slices. Transfer to a deep pot and add enough water to cover. Cook until each slice softens.

Remove from the heat and drain. Allow it to cool for a while.

Meanwhile, repeat the process with broccoli. They take about 10 minutes to soften. Combine the potato with broccoli, season with some salt and olive oil.

This recipe is almost impossible without garlic. 1 crushed garlic clove will be enough. Combine it with olive oil, add 1 tablespoon of finely chopped parsley and pour over vegetables.

Nutrition information per serving: Kcal: 451, Protein: 26.1g, Carbs: 7.4g, Fats: 36.2g

52.   Fresh Carrot Risotto with Prunes

Ingredients:

1 cup of brown rice, pre-cooked

2 tbsp. extra virgin olive oil

2 medium-sized carrots, grated

1 small tomato, peeled and finely chopped

1 tsp of vegetable seasoning mix

1 medium-sized onion, peeled and chopped

½ cup of prunes, chopped

Preparation:

In a deep pot, bring 3 cups of water to a boiling point. Add rice, reduce the heat to minimum, and cook until the water evaporates. Remove from the heat.

Heat up the olive oil in a frying pan over a medium-high temperature. Add onion and stir-fry until translucent. Now add tomato, apricots, and vegetable seasoning mix. Cook for five more minutes and add rice. Stir well to combine.

Top with prunes and serve.

Nutrition information per serving: Kcal: 311, Protein: 4.8g, Carbs: 56.2g, Fats: 8.4g

53. Cashew Cream and Broccoli Stew

Ingredients:

2 oz of fresh broccoli

A handful of fresh parsley, finely chopped

1 tsp of dry thyme, ground

1 tbsp of fresh lemon juice

¼ tsp of chili pepper, ground

3 tbsp of olive oil

1 tbsp of cashew cream

Preparation:

Place the broccoli in a deep pot and pour enough water to cover. Bring it to a boil and cook until tender. Remove from the heat and drain.

Transfer to a food processor. Add fresh parsley, thyme, and about ½ cup of water. Pulse until smooth mixture. Return to a pot and add some more water. Bring it to a boil and cook for several minutes, over a minimum temperature.

Stir in some olive oil and cashew cream, sprinkle with ground chili pepper and add fresh lemon juice. Serve warm.

Nutrition information per serving: Kcal: 72 Protein: 12.2g, Carbs: 15.8g, Fats: 8.3g

54.   Tuna Pasta

Ingredients:

1 cup of minced tuna

½ cup of homemade cashew cream

2 cups of rice flour macaroni

1 tsp of sea salt

1 tsp of olive oil

1 tbsp of canola oil

Few olives for decoration (optional)

Preparation:

Pour 3 cups of water in a pot. Bring it to boil and add macaroni and salt. Boil macaroni for about 3 minutes (rice flour macaroni take less time to cook). You can also use the package instructions to cook macaroni, if you're not sure. Remove from heat and drain.

In a bowl, combine tuna with homemade cashew cream. Mash well with a fork.

In a large saucepan, combine the olive oil with canola oil. Heat up over a medium temperature and add tuna mixture.

Fry for about 15-20 minutes stirring occasionally. Add macaroni and mix well. Cover the saucepan and allow macaroni to heat up. Serve warm with some olives.

Nutrition information per serving: Kcal: 224, Protein: 33.2g, Carbs: 44.3g, Fats: 12.5g

55.   Rosemary Salmon

Ingredients:

2 lbs of fresh salmon, sliced into 1 inch slices

1 cup of extra-virgin olive oil

3 tbsp of lemon juice, freshly squeezed

1 tbsp of fresh rosemary, finely chopped

1 tsp of dry oregano, ground

1 dry bay leaf, crushed

1 tsp of salt

1 tbsp of cayenne pepper, ground

Preparation:

Combine the olive oil with lemon juice, chopped rosemary, dry oregano, bay leaf, salt, and cayenne pepper. Stir well to combine.

Using a kitchen brush, spread this mixture over the salmon sliced. Let it stand for about 10-15 minutes.

Meanwhile, preheat the grill pan over a medium-high heat. Grill the salmon slices for 3 minutes, on each side.

Nutrition information per serving: Kcal: 261, Protein: 26g Carbs: 0.2g Fats: 16.1g

ADDITIONAL TITLES FROM THIS AUTHOR

70 Effective Meal Recipes to Prevent and Solve Being Overweight: Burn Fat Fast by Using Proper Dieting and Smart Nutrition

By

Joe Correa CSN

48 Acne Solving Meal Recipes: The Fast and Natural Path to Fixing Your Acne Problems in Less Than 10 Days!

By

Joe Correa CSN

41 Alzheimer's Preventing Meal Recipes: Reduce or Eliminate Your Alzheimer's Condition in 30 Days or Less!

By

Joe Correa CSN

70 Effective Breast Cancer Meal Recipes: Prevent and Fight Breast Cancer with Smart Nutrition and Powerful Foods

By

Joe Correa CSN

www.ingramcontent.com/pod-product-compliance
Lightning Source LLC
Chambersburg PA
CBHW030245030426
42336CB00009B/257